RSI

Repetitive
Strain Injury

RSI

Repetitive
Strain Injury

REPETITIVE STRAIN INJURY, CARPAL TUNNEL
SYNDROME AND OTHER OFFICE NUMBERS

Wendy Chalmers Mill
MCSP, SRP, Dip RGRT

Thorsons
An Imprint of HarperCollins*Publishers*

Thorsons
An Imprint of HarperCollins*Publishers*
77–85 Fulham Palace Road,
Hammersmith, London W6 8JB
1160 Battery Street,
San Francisco, California 94111-1213

Published by Thorsons 1994
1 3 5 7 9 10 8 6 4 2

© Wendy Chalmers Mill 1994

Wendy Chalmers Mill asserts the moral right to
be identified as the author of this work

A catalogue record for this book
is available from the British Library

ISBN 0 7225 2919 8

Printed in Great Britain by
HarperCollinsManufacturing Glasgow

Illustrations by Peter Cox

Contents

Introduction

The rapid growth of information technology has transformed the working environment, and most of us find ourselves spending a lot more of our time sitting in front of a computer screen. Not only is this the case for nearly all jobs, but it applies to schools as well—and a computer at home is also now the norm rather than the exception, not to mention the proliferation of game consoles and what amounts almost to a mass addiction to computer games amongst children.

Since computers are set to play a progressively greater part in our daily lives it is important that we understand what implications there may be to our health from their sustained use. Considerable publicity has been given to one particular set of problems associated with constant keyboard work, and that is overuse disorders—referred to as repetitive strain injury (RSI), and also as occupational overuse syndrome or cumulative trauma disorder. Very little has been published about its possible causes, and even less about preventive measures. In my practice as a Chartered Physiotherapist I have specialized in treating, curing and preventing RSI, and the practical advice that is given in this book derives from my extensive experience in rehabilitating RSI sufferers.

The patients I have treated have often been young—at the beginning of their working lives—and they have been under a great deal of mental as well as physical pressure. Although it has been my job to deal with the physical side of their condition, it has been impossible to ignore the psychological effects that RSI has. Some of my patients had begun to think that there was nothing that could be done to help them. Because the medical profession has tended to show a lack of awareness of this particular problem, they feared that they had contracted some mysterious illness which could not be diagnosed, let alone be treated.

I have generally suggested professional counselling in such cases. This is not because I wish to perpetuate the myth that RSI is a purely psychological illness. It is a very real physical condition caused by the maltreatment of the body's chemistry and mechanics, and it is wrong to under-estimate the impact this painful condition can have on the state of mind of a sufferer.

There is really no mystery about RSI. It is inevitable that by sitting static in front of a computer terminal, hammering away at the keyboard for sustained periods day after day under stress and in robot fashion, we run the risk of fatigue and injury. It is all too easy to ignore the early signs of muscle ache, tension or pain, but we do so at our peril. Continued abuse of our bodies will only add to the problem and make recovery that much harder to achieve.

The treatment which I have used with considerable success involves individually designed stretch programmes designed to elongate the contracted tissues and improve the biomechanical/chemical functions, and the duration of treatment depends on the patient and the degree of damage done prior to treatment being sought.

The fact is, though, that the problem need never occur if sensible preventive action is taken. It should be recognized that we are not robots in a production line. Workloads should be realistic, with regular breaks, short stretches, intermittent changes of task and properly designed work stations. If we ignore these simple measures we run the risk of damaging our health and losing our livelihoods. I hope what I say in this book will point sufferers in the right direction and will enable others to avoid ever contracting RSI.

What is RSI?

The condition commonly referred to as repetitive strain injury is also known by a variety of other names, such as: cumulative trauma disorder; occupational cervical brachial disorder, overuse syndrome, repetitive strain syndrome and work-related upper limb disorder.

Cumulative trauma disorder is what the Americans call RSI, and it does seem to describe the problem more accurately. The implication of the term RSI (more a product of the media than a medical expression) is that the cause is solely repetition, whilst in fact it is not nearly so simplistic. There are three main contributory factors—static posture, overuse and stress. Together these have the potential to cause a major disruption of the nervous system, tendons, muscles and joints. However, since the name RSI has, for all its shortcomings, become popular usage I have chosen to continue using it in this book. I ask readers to bear in mind, though, that cumulative trauma disorder, and the rather unwieldy term work-related upper limb disorder convey more precisely what we are talking about.

STATIC POSTURE

Basic Physiology

The evolution of human beings as two-legged creatures has resulted in modifications in the body's musculature to permit us to stand as we do today. The muscles involved are what I call 'anti-gravity muscles', and they are largely those muscles found around the spine and in our legs. These anti-gravity muscles are constantly contracted and statically loaded to bear the weight of our bodies in the standing position. However, the body is designed for movement while keeping its skeletal shape intact.

For thousands of years humans have used their bodies consistent with the way they have evolved, spending their days in the open air, mostly walking or running in an upright posture, first as hunter, then as herdsman and farmer. Prolonged periods of sitting down were not part of the evolutionary design, yet the development of modern society has called for most of us to spend our days doing just that, either at desks, counters, check-outs, benches, conveyor belts—and in more cases than not there is today a computer screen in front of us.

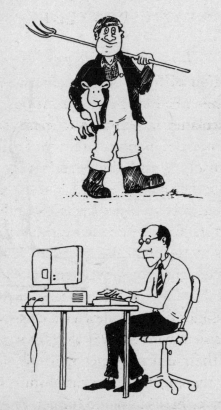

The difference between moving and static jobs

The pace at which these new demands have come to be made of our bodies has far outstripped the speed of evolutionary change. You could say that our brains have developed quicker than our

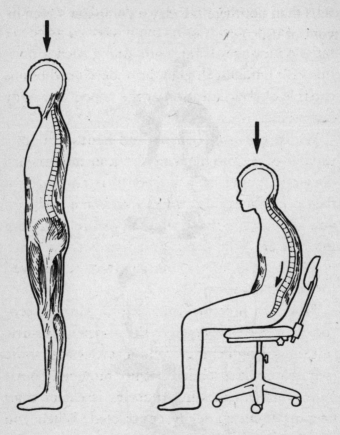

The difference between muscles used when standing and sitting

bodies! Think about the way you sit at a keyboard. Think how this differs from the way you stand, walk and move. Try to imagine a monkey sitting static on a chair looking at a screen. I suggest that it would fidget and lose interest very quickly as its brain received its body's fatigue messages from maintaining such a position. We humans, though, have developed brains capable of concentration at the expense of body awareness.

Whilst our arms, wrists and hands are quite capable of performing many intricate movements, constant typing on a keyboard is an abuse of their capabilities. Also, when you sit at a keyboard you adopt a totally new *fixed* posture. Different muscles are now being asked to become 'anti-gravity muscles'. These muscles have not evolved for this function—yet!

There are three basic muscle functions: concentric (meaning shortening of the muscle), eccentric (meaning lengthening of the muscle) and static (where muscle is loaded but not moving). Shortening and lengthening muscles is easier than keeping them statically contracted. When you sit at a keyboard you are keeping muscles which should be moving in a fixed or statically contracted position against the force of gravity. Muscles become fatigued and start aching as the blood supply slows and fails to deliver oxygen to clear the waste products from the system.

Continually fixed positions can lead to contracted statically loaded muscles, constricted blood vessels, immobile joints and tethered/-compressed nerves, causing neuritis (inflammation of the nerves) or neuralgia (pain in the nerves).

It will help in the understanding of what a tethered/compressed nerve is if you imagine a hosepipe running through a garden. While it runs along the lawn there are no problems, but if the hosepipe has to negotiate a right-angled bend around a house there will be two effects: where the hose bends there may be compression and localized damage; and there may be a disruption to the output or distribution of the water in the hosepipe. So it is in the body—when a nerve travels from your neck to your fingers directly down a straight arm, where there are no constrictions, there is little problem. However, if instead the nerve travels through dense fibrous tissue, elevated shoulders, bent elbows and wrists, its function may be inhibited and there may be compression or tension in the nerve structures.

The symptoms of static posture are frequently first felt in the muscles and nerves. You may feel tense (especially around the neck and shoulders), with aching muscles, eye strain, tension headaches and low back pain. Your breathing can become shallow, clumsiness develops and general fatigue sets in. The constricted blood vessels and slowed circulation may possibly result in swollen, mottled and blue hands. The nerve compression, or tethering, can give very intense non-specific pain, such as sharp shooting pains, tingling, numbness and pins-and-needles.

The spinal shape and posture can also have an effect on nerves and muscles, reducing blood flow, causing compression to structures centred around the spine. This may provoke symptoms of sweating, swelling, colour and temperature changes.

The symptoms caused by lack of movement can occur at any time, anywhere. You do not necessarily have to be sitting at a keyboard; you could be knitting, or playing an instrument, or lying in bed.

OVERUSE

The second contributory factor is overuse, or repetition. This is where the term RSI (repetitive strain injury) comes in, and in its purest form RSI confines itself to specific areas of trauma injuries such as lateral epicondylitis (tennis-elbow), medial epicondylitis (golfer's elbow), tenosynovitis, tendonitis, carpal-tunnel syndrome, supraspinatus tendonitis, de Quervain's disease and ganglions.

Epicondylitis
This is damage either side of the elbow at the junction where all the extensor (tennis elbow) and flexor (golfer's elbow) muscles join on to the bone.

Tenosynovitis
Inflammation of the synovial sheath surrounding a tendon.

Tendonitis
Inflammation of a tendon.

Carpal-tunnel syndrome

Compression on the median nerve in the carpal tunnel and a reduction in blood flow, leading to inflammation and pain at the wrist.

Supraspinatus tendonitis

Inflammation of the supraspinatus muscle in the shoulder.

de Quervain's disease

This is a tendon tunnel syndrome involving inflammation of the tendon sheath in the thumb and down the same side of the wrist.

Ganglions

Cystic swellings which generally take the form of a small painless lump around a joint or tendon sheath, most commonly found on the upper part of the wrist.

Regular keyboard users are particularly prone to the above conditions.

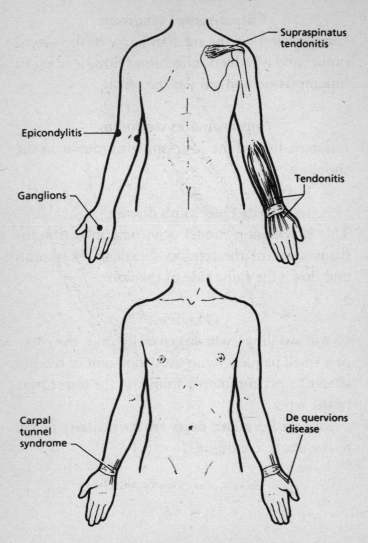

Areas of localized injuries

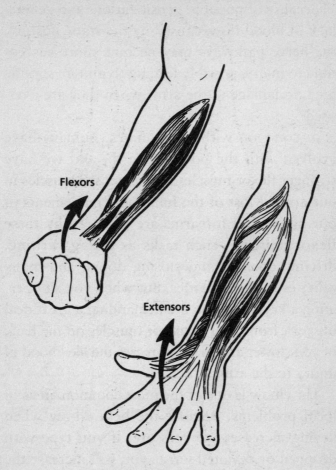

Flexor and extensor muscles

11

Because of possible 'sensitization' and general lack of blood flow, caused by the static posture, the nerve pathways may become more susceptible to injury, possibly leading to a more specific area of damage in the arms when they are overused.

In common with all primates, humans have evolved with the power to grip, and we have stronger flexor muscles than extensor muscles in our arms. Most of the functional movements of our hands and forearms are powered by these flexor muscles—such tasks as eating, writing, driving, opening and closing doors, and many other everyday activities. But when you sit operating a keyboard you are demanding a great deal of work from your extensor muscles on the back of your lower arm. This increases the likelihood of injury to the arms.

The elbow is one of the most common areas of local problems, because the bent elbow when keying increases the pressure. If you type with dropped or deviated wrists you will increase the likelihood of the development of carpal-tunnel syndrome as the pressure is greater inside the carpal tunnel. The condition can be further aggravated by restricted blood flow and possible nerve sensitivity arising from static posture, which in turn limit the self-healing process.

Pain from this local injury will increase your stress level, which will lead on to yet more tension in your already overstrained muscles.

STRESS

Learning to cope with stress begins with self-awareness. Many chemical changes occur in your body when you are presented with a challenging or exciting situation. These are to prepare you for whatever action is necessary. This is short-term stress, and the symptoms will disappear after the challenge has been met and overcome.

Messages sent from the brain have a direct effect on body functions. Stress can be positive and motivational, but if it is not managed the body starts to suffer the consequences. Imagine tomorrow you are going for an interview. Your body reacts to the stimulus by releasing chemicals which 'gee' your body up, and you may become anxious and tense. After the interview your body chemistry normalizes.

If you had an interview every other day, the

chemicals which are released would never normalize (unless you were able to manage the stimulus) and they would keep your body in a state of constant tension—this is unmanaged stress.

However, if you are sitting working in a noisy office, with phones ringing and people talking, as you try to concentrate on a myriad things while confronted by the challenge of deadlines to meet, your body is forced into a continuous stress response—unmanaged stress—with little or no chance to calm down and normalize.

The cumulative effect of this can be a general increase in body tension, headaches, backache, ulcers, indigestion, constipation or diarrhoea, blood pressure changes, loss of appetite, skin problems and heart conditions, including palpitations.

These stress symptoms can only increase the effects of any pressure from static posture and localized repetitive strain (or overuse disorder), thus leading to a vicious circle.

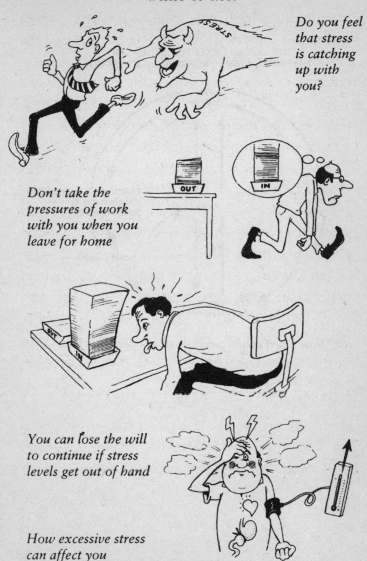

Do you feel that stress is catching up with you?

Don't take the pressures of work with you when you leave for home

You can lose the will to continue if stress levels get out of hand

How excessive stress can affect you

THE VICIOUS CIRCLE HYPOTHESIS OF
THE INITIAL SYMPTOMS OF W.R.U.L.D.S (RSI)

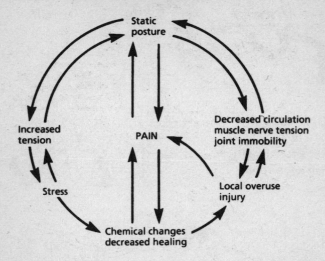

Flow chart of the physiological effects of stress

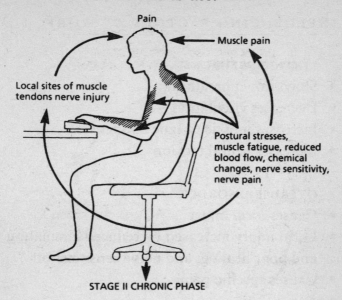

Pain

Muscle pain

Local sites of muscle tendons nerve injury

Postural stresses, muscle fatigue, reduced blood flow, chemical changes, nerve sensitivity, nerve pain

STAGE II CHRONIC PHASE

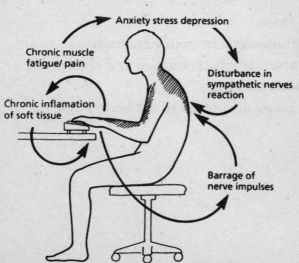

Anxiety stress depression

Chronic muscle fatigue/ pain

Disturbance in sympathetic nerves reaction

Chronic inflamation of soft tissue

Barrage of nerve impulses

INFLUENCING FACTORS AT WORK

STATIC POSTURE
- Slows down breathing
- Decreases circulation
- Increases muscle fatigue and tension
- Increases neural tension

OVERUSE DISORDER
- Causes *local* injury
- Local injury increased by reduced circulation and poor healing, and nerve sensitization
- Causes specific pain

STRESS
- Stimulates a hormone reaction
- Increases muscle tension and changes to body chemistry
- Causes disruption to the body's systems

Preventive Measures

The introduction of computers into the workplace is thought to mean fewer people are capable of doing more work in half the time. Surely no one would go to the expense of installing such expensive and complicated technology unless they thought there was an end gain. Unfortunately, there can also be a potential end loss—the damage it can do to our health.

It is not my aim to frighten you off ever touching a keyboard again, and my purpose in this book is to take a positive attitude towards RSI and how to prevent it. However, we should not forget the risk of injury from using modern day equipment incorrectly. Both employers and employees have to be aware of the risk—as it takes both sides working together to prevent it. There is no point in workers conscientiously carrying out preventive routines if the boss stands there and glares every time they take a break;

just as there is no point in an employer buying ergonomically designed chairs only for employees to perch on the edge of their seats.

In proofing ourselves against RSI we have to look at two aspects—one is our work environment and the other is the correct use of our bodies. The next chapter deals with the environmental aspect, and in this chapter I concentrate on what *you* can do to make sure you don't join the ranks of RSI sufferers.

All three of the contributory causes of RSI— static posture, overuse and stress—are directly influenced by the way you use your body and mind. Only you can know what your body is capable of, and only you can be aware of what your body is telling you. If you leave work every night with a headache, an aching neck and stiff shoulders, arriving home so tired that you can do little else but slump in front of the TV, something is clearly not right!

STATIC POSTURE

Do not dismiss your aches and pains and lethargy as normal—you *can* do something about it. Of course, all of us have periods in our working lives when we are particularly under pressure, and are both expected and prepared to work for long hours. This is going to make us more fatigued than usual, but a few simple stretches can go a long way to increasing blood flow, reducing body tension and general fatigue (see page 25).

Improving your general fitness will enhance the quality of your life, and will fortify your resistance to everyday pressures—those pressures that can contribute to the development of RSI if you let them. Mental and physical exhaustion, whether real or perceived, are the first symptoms that your body is being put under more stress and strain than is good for it. Take stock of the way you feel. Are you enjoying your work, or do you arrive each morning already feeling tired and tense? A few simple actions on your part can make a great deal of difference to the quality of your life, and you will probably find that the quality of your work also improves, along with your spirits.

How to Avoid Static Posture

An airline hostess was asked by a passenger why she wasn't smiling that famous air-hostess smile. 'OK,' she said, 'you smile.' The passenger did so —a nice cheerful grin. 'Right,' said the air-hostess, 'now hold that for eight hours.' This illustrates what is meant by fixed static posture. Of course, you would notice if you had to smile for eight hours a day, your face would get tired and your muscles would ache.

Have you ever thought how you hold tension in other parts of your body for hours and hours each day? Have you ever considered what you are doing to yourself? In your mind, briefly draw a comparison between a person sitting in front of a VDU for eight hours and a monkey freely leaping and swinging through the jungle. Ask yourself which body could function for longer. You might not realize it, but you are quite likely to be sitting in the same position, looking at the same object for hour upon hour, a bit like an adult version of the children's game 'musical statues'. Remember, your body is designed to move, and movement encourages a healthy body.

Make a conscious effort to get up out of your

seat more often. Although you may not think so, one of the easiest things you can introduce into your office routine is a screen break. Do not be fooled by the nagging thought that you do not have time. A screen break can be from one minute to five minutes. If you totalled up all the minutes of wasted thoughts throughout the day there would be plenty of time to take adequate and conscious breaks from the keyboard. Make sure that at least once every hour you take a break

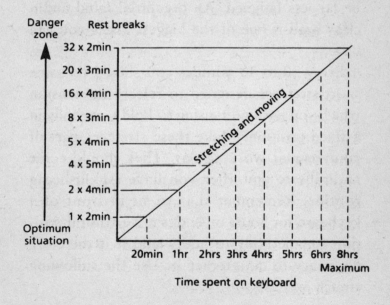

Graph of rest breaks

23

from your computer screen. The more intensive the task, the more rest breaks you need.

During your break, get up, walk around and do some stretching. Perhaps go to get a cup of coffee. Get yourself away from your desk and refocus your eyes on something different. Taking these few minutes away from your desk every so often gives you a chance to get a different perspective on what you are doing. It will mean that you get more work done as your brain and muscles will be far less fatigued. An organized mind and a clear head is one of the biggest assets you can have.

Every 20 to 30 minutes you should do some short stretches designed to release the tension which you have been using to hold your body in a fixed position. Make these stretches part of your regular working day. They should come naturally to you after you have established a routine. Remember that to sit in front of a keyboard for hours on end is not a natural position for the body to adopt and it is therefore necessary to counteract it. Use the following stretch exercises.

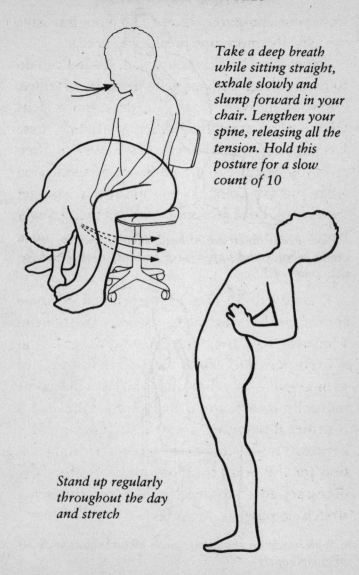

Take a deep breath while sitting straight, exhale slowly and slump forward in your chair. Lengthen your spine, releasing all the tension. Hold this posture for a slow count of 10

Stand up regularly throughout the day and stretch

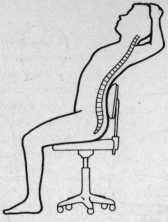

a: Place hands on crown of head, keeping chin in, gently stretch elbows and upper back towards roof. Hold for slow count of 3

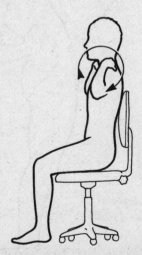

b: With hands on shoulders, circle elbows backwards 10 times vigorously

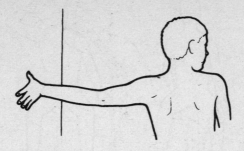

c: Push shoulder down. Place palm of hand on wall and gently straighten elbow. DO NOT PUSH INTO PAIN. Hold for slow count of 3

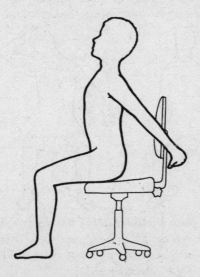

d: Clasp hands and keeping back/neck straight raise arms backwards and look towards roof. Hold for count of 3

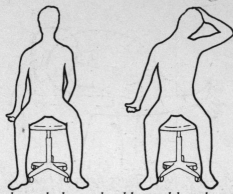

e: (i) Gently push down shoulder and lengthen arm, pull hand back with palm towards front with elbow straight. (ii) If there is no pain, gently stretch head away. Hold for count of 3

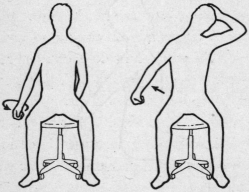

f: (i) Gently push shoulder down and lengthen arm. Make a fist with thumb tucked in hand and rotate arm. (ii) If there is no pain, gently elevate arm away from body and stretch head away. Hold for count of 3

NOTE: *In exercises c, e and f you may experience some tingling. DO NOT push/stretch further than this sensation*

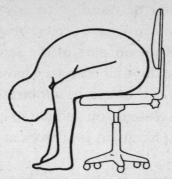

g: Slump in chair, lengthen the spine. Hold for count of 5

Once every hour try to stand up and take a longer break away from your work. It might be an opportunity to get some fresh air and re-acquaint yourself with the world outside. Don't feel guilty about it—you are not 'skiving off'. Being away from your computer keyboard also gives you a chance to take a 'mind break'. During this time try to think of something pleasant—lying in the sun on a beautiful beach or swimming in a warm blue lagoon.

Perhaps one way of making sure you take regular breaks is to set an alarm clock or stop watch. If you sit next to someone you can synchronize your work patterns and share the same breaks. Perhaps when the phone rings you make a point of standing to answer it. Some computer systems have screen break reminders which flash up on part of the screen every so often. These do not necessarily have to interrupt your work, as they can be unobtrusive, and they are there to remind you and not to increase stress by causing a hiccup in your work as you strive to finish a job.

Remember that after two hours of intense keyboard work, mistakes become more frequent—increased spelling errors etc. Taking short 2–3 minutes breaks will reduce your errors and increase your efficiency.

As you get into the swing of taking regular breaks they will easily become part of your routine. The last thing you want is for them to become an intrusion on your work and thereby increase stress levels. It is, though, hard to remember to take breaks without a mechanical reminder, particularly if you are the intense type who gets deeply involved with work—the type particularly prone to RSI!

Old habits die hard, and you might be a little dubious about these suggestions—your employer could be even less happy—but regular screen breaks and short stretches will go a long way towards making sure that you never suffer from incapacitating RSI. If you are happy and healthy at work you will be more productive and the company's efficiency will also improve.

During the time that you are hard at work, find a moment or two to occasionally remind yourself that you are indeed a person, not an extension of your computer, and that it is unnatural to be sitting for an indefinite period of time. If at all possible, try to rotate your tasks throughout your day. If you have three things to do that are sedentary, and another two which involve walking about, intersperse the sitting with the moving. Sometimes this may not be possible, but it is certainly worth thinking about. New government legislation brought out in January 1993 encourages employers to be aware of the value of task rotation and screen breaks.

It is important also to be aware of your eyes. Remember your eyes are worked by muscles. They will fatigue and weaken just like any other muscle. Looking at your screen for hours on end will eventually take its toll, and they need to be 'stretched' by being allowed to focus on the middle and far distance from time to time.

A good employer should encourage workers to

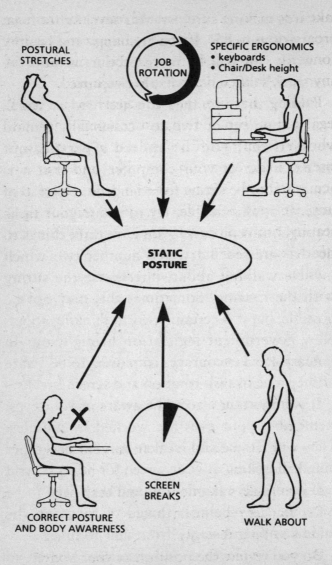

POSTURAL
STRETCHES

JOB
ROTATION

SPECIFIC ERGONOMICS
• keyboards
• Chair/Desk height

STATIC
POSTURE

CORRECT POSTURE
AND BODY AWARENESS

SCREEN
BREAKS

WALK ABOUT

take screen breaks and should introduce training programmes to educate staff on the correct use of computer equipment so that the occurrence of any work-related disorders is minimized.

Publicity has been given recently to successful legal actions brought against companies by staff who have contracted RSI, so it is in a company's interest to do everything possible to prevent any occupational injury. At the same time the employer will enjoy the benefit of employing a healthy, happy and positive staff and all that that means to productivity levels.

Answer 'yes' or 'no' to the following questions to see how much static posture is affecting you.

STATIC POSTURE CHECKLIST   YES/NO

- Are you aware that you sit correctly?
- Do you sit for longer than one hour?
- Is your posture fixed doing the same thing?
- Do you feel a constant ache in your neck and shoulders?
- Do you suffer frequent headaches?
- Do you get regular backache?
- Do you fatigue easily?
- Do you review the position of your body?

I say again, you are a person not a machine. Unlike a machine, you cannot go on working non-stop. It is a simple physiological fact that your body can only take so much. Your nerves, joints, ligaments, muscles, and tendons are all vulnerable to overuse. You wouldn't expect your legs to be able to carry you for hundreds of miles non-stop, so why do you think you can push other parts of your body beyond the limit with no adverse effects?

OVERUSE

Unfortunately for our poor bodies, computer technology has evolved more quickly than our own internal evolutionary software. Maybe, in a couple of million years from now, we will have evolved into a new super race anatomically developed to utilize the forearm functionally, and capable of looking at a computer monitor for eight hours a day without a break, and of sitting in one position all day without getting up to walk around—all without adverse effect!

Until that time we are going to have to accept our limitations and live within them. On a practical everyday level, that could well mean reducing your workload to eliminate the risk of RSI. Taking regular rest breaks will not only help reduce the effects of static posture, it will also prevent local repetitive strain problems. Specific stretching and localized massage will increase the circulation to the areas at risk of overuse. Try to vary your workload and rotate your tasks. Tell yourself and your boss that you cannot work flat out all the time. Don't take on more than you can cope with; it will only increase your error rate and cause you to have to repeat work.

A reduction of the workload on your body could be achieved by just a little office reorganization. It might be that someone else could take over some of your keyboard work in exchange for your periodically doing a different task. This is in both your interest and that of your employer, as the company will not be getting the best from its workforce if time off for work-related illness is at high levels. It is better that you both recognize that there is something wrong and begin to act on it straight away, and as with all things it is preferable to be pro-active rather than reactive—in other words taking preventive action before the event rather than after. Early reporting of symptoms will save your health and save company time and money in the long term.

It is important that your employer is aware of new health and safety legislations. If not, a copy of the regulations can be obtained from the government Health and Safety Executive. Assume that your employer will be interested in this, and remember that a healthy workforce is as much in the company's interest as it is in yours. You can talk to your employer, leave a copy of this book lying around, or get a physiotherapist or ergonomist to talk about the risks. Whatever you do, don't let it fall on deaf ears. Point out that it is not usually lazy or workshy people who get RSI, and that ignoring this potential problem is not going to make it go away.

The condition is a very painful and debilitating one, which in extreme circumstances can cripple you for the rest of your life, and positive action can stop unnecessary suffering.

Good management = healthy staff = increased productivity = improved company efficiency.

Answer 'yes' or 'no' to the following questions to see how much you need to change your ways.

OVERUSE/REPETITION CHECKLIST YES/NO

- Do you take screen breaks?
- Do you have task rotation?
- Do you stand up and walk around frequently?
- Do you rest your forearms when not typing?
- Do you relax, especially your shoulders?
- Do you focus your eyes on different distances?
- Do you hammer the keyboard?
- Do you take active deep breaths?
- Do you review your work station and the position of your body?

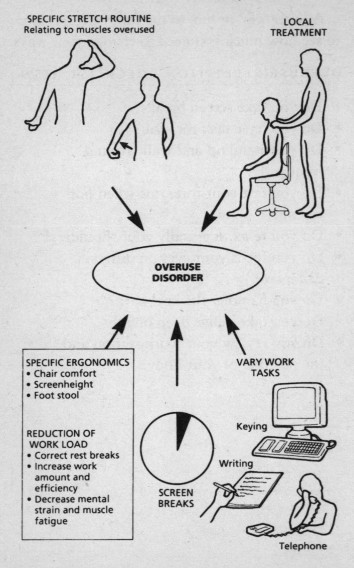

SPECIFIC STRETCH ROUTINE
Relating to muscles overused

LOCAL
TREATMENT

OVERUSE
DISORDER

SPECIFIC ERGONOMICS
• Chair comfort
• Screenheight
• Foot stool

REDUCTION OF
WORK LOAD
• Correct rest breaks
• Increase work
  amount and
  efficiency
• Decrease mental
  strain and muscle
  fatigue

VARY WORK
TASKS

Keying

Writing

SCREEN
BREAKS

Telephone

STRESS AND HOW TO PREVENT IT

There is no shortage of articles on stress in popular magazines, and most of us would presume to understand what stress is and what it means. However, in my experience most people have absolutely no idea of how much stress or tension their bodies hold. How long, for instance, does it take you to get really annoyed in a traffic jam? How furious do you get when the person in front of you at the Post Office counter decides to pay for his TV licence in 50p pieces and then accidentally delays things further by dropping them on the floor? Such frustrations can quite soon turn us into seething fire-breathing dragons, resulting in twisted knots of tension in our bodies.

Take a look at what really annoys you. If it is sitting in your car in a traffic jam, why not see if you can travel by other means—letting the bus or the train take the strain. If you live close to work perhaps you could cycle there. If lunchtime shopping proves too much, then do it some other time—most supermarkets are now open after office hours and many are open all weekend. Try not to let tension creep into your body in circumstances over which you have no control. Dwell on other thoughts which induce a feeling of calm.

Whilst at school we took regular breaks, generally a milk break in the morning, a lunch break and then perhaps another break in the afternoon. Somewhere along the line we have forgotten about them. Coffee breaks and lunch breaks serve a purpose—allowing us time to recuperate—so use them. Don't just sit at your desk munching a sandwich as you continue to bash away at your keyboard. Perhaps you could find some time to go swimming in your lunch break. Some companies have keep-fit facilities on the premises, or they have an arrangement with a local health club. It is in your interest to use them. Many local sports halls hold 40-minute lunch hour exercise classes. You never know, you might start to enjoy them!

You may find this extreme, but remember that the pressures of modern day living cause us to ask far more from our bodies. To compensate for this some time must be given back to your body. Whatever you do, try to get out of the office, even if it's only for 10 or 20 minutes. Go outside, remind yourself that there is a world beyond the four walls you work within. If you go out for a drink with your colleagues, try to talk about something other than work.

From time to time allow yourself a sneaky 10 seconds just to take stock. Even if you end up thinking about what you are going to do at the weekend, or whose birthday card you have to buy at lunchtime, this encourages short mind breaks. I'm not suggesting that you pay less attention to your work.

Relaxation

It can be seen from today's many stress-related illnesses that relaxation is crucial, but learning to relax is not easy. A simplified way of describing 'relaxation' is the lengthening of the body. There are two types of relaxation; passive and active.

Passive relaxation is when you unconsciously switch off from the stimulus which causes the stress—you might watch TV, or go out for a walk, or even go to the pub!

Active relaxation is when you consciously focus into your body and relieve tension with different techniques, such as yoga, meditation, t'ai chi, flotation tanks, or breathing techniques.

Most of you reading this book will have been imbued with a Protestant work ethic at a very early age. This may have been very good for your career, but perhaps not so good for your health. There is nothing wrong with working hard, most of us frequently quite enjoy it, but do think about how much of your day is spent unproductively. This is in effect dead time as you are not using it for work or rest.

Why not get a piece of paper and write down what you do in a day? Look at the list and you will probably find some time you have to yourself. What do you do with this time? Do you enjoy the way you use it? Could you use the time to better effect? Is there space there when you could take 30 minutes to do some regular exercise? It might seem like an effort to take the dog out for a walk after a hard day in the office, but it will do you good.

Perhaps enrol at a yoga class, or try training in Alexander Technique. Other possibilities are, as above, meditation, hypnotherapy, aromatherapy, massage or a few sessions in a flotation tank. Any one of these will not only help you to relax your body and mind, they will also help you to become more aware of your body and your tension. Relaxation will also help you re-learn how to breathe!

Breathing

Most of us breathe badly without realizing it. We don't allow our diaphragms (the drumskin under our ribcage) to move properly. We sit cramped up at a desk and breathe little shallow breaths with the top of our lungs. It's no accident that we breathe a sigh of relief. Breathing properly and thoughtfully is good for us. It relaxes our face muscles, it relaxes our bodies and our minds. Taking a deep breath is like filling your car up with fuel—we fill our bodies up with oxygen, flooding our muscles, stopping fatigue and keeping ourselves in good running order.

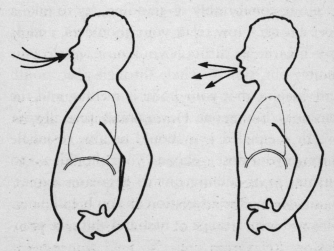

Practise breathing properly.

Another way to breathe is not to make a conscious effort to breathe in, but to think of something that makes you smile. With your mouth turned up, allow your lower jaw and tongue to drop, and breathe out saying 'aahhh' until your lungs are empty. Do this once or twice whenever you feel particularly stressed. It can be quite difficult to discipline yourself to this exercise, but you will feel better for it. Thinking about breathing in this active way for five minutes each day helps decrease the feeling of tension and anxiety, muscle ache, chest pain and pins and needles.

Sitting comfortably or standing, try to take a deep breath. Now relax your shoulders, and as you breathe in through your nose, push your tummy out, slowly exhale through your mouth and imagine that your body is melting and the tension is drifting out. Having made sure all your breath is exhaled you should be able to inhale through your nose, relaxing your shoulders and pushing your tummy out to a greater extent. Again, feeling the relaxation as you breathe out. This will seem strange at first and will take practice.

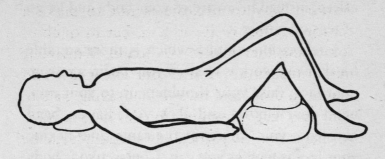

Lie comfortably on back with knee and back of head supported. Breathe deeply feeling body lengthening and relaxing

Lying on the floor in the above position, start deep breathing—in through your nose and out through your mouth. With each inward breath feel your body warming as you draw in colours of red or orange. With each outward breath think of expelling cold colours—blues and greens—and let them melt away along with tension. Focus on any tension and ache.

Concentrating on your body, feeling it getting heavier and sinking into the floor; slowly and rhythmically continue to breathe deeply, bringing warmth into your body and breathing out the cold, and let the tension drift out of your muscles. As you relax more completely your body should become heavier. Do not permit yourself to fall

45

asleep, instead be aware of your body and let go of tension within it.

A relaxation routine which is more suitable for doing at work is to sit in your chair, screw up your face, raise your shoulders up to your ears, bend your elbows and claw your hands, bend and tense your knees, at the same time flexing your feet as high as you can. Contract your body into as tight a ball as you can and hold it rigid for a slow count of five. Then release everything, breathing out at the same time. Return to your correct sitting posture and reassure your colleagues that you have not gone crazy!

Another, perhaps obvious, way to reduce tension is to wrap up warm in cold weather. Insubstantial coats and too thin soles on your shoes can leave you with tight shoulders, clenched fists and aching legs as you brace yourself against the elements. Wear clothes you feel comfortable in, and when it's cold layer them over each other.

Coping with Anxiety

Home anxieties can be another stress factor. Even when you think you leave them behind to go to work, you are often in a more tense state when you arrive. Going through a 'bad patch' with your partner or having a difficult time with a rebellious adolescent, a bereavement or worrying about an ageing relative will all take their toll of you, both mentally and physically.

Occasionally, in my experience with patients, anxieties outside of work have induced or triggered problems associated with keyboard activities. Someone may have been using a keyboard for 40 years and, even though their body is used to typing, their stress levels have suddenly increased, bringing on physical problems.

Remember the physical causes of RSI:

STATIC POSTURE
REPETITION
STRESS

It only takes an increase in one of the factors to upset the apple cart.

There are no quick and easy answers to helping you overcome this sort of worry, but you must try not to let your body absorb your mental stress. Personal trauma can lead to a greater susceptibility to illness and whatever negative thoughts you harbour may eventually show themselves in painful physical symptoms, so it is important to put them in perspective and not allow them to affect your health.

ORGANIZATION

Think about your office and the way you work. Is your desk organized and tidy? Do you have a list of objectives, and do you prioritize them? Are you putting yourself under unnecessary strain? Do you stumble over problems or conquer the challenges?

If you live your office life in a continual whirl with a chaotic work space, your tension and stress levels will naturally increase. Take some time each day to give yourself an overview of what you are doing. With some sense of proportion and a set of priorities you can feel much more positive about what you have already achieved and what you can go on to do. Set yourself small goals. Don't get gloomy and let a cloud envelop your work. Leave the office with a sense of achievement.

A happy workplace goes a long way towards reducing stress levels. Inspirational leadership and good management will result in people coping happily and effectively with a considerable workload. It is not new technology that gets the best results, it is the people who operate the equipment. If the motivation is there, all of us are capable of things we never dreamed possible. Unfortunately, this is not always recognized and there are many places where disillusioned and downcast staff are not performing at their best.

I urge employers to give thought to ways in which their staff can be made happier and more comfortable, and I don't mean pay rises. The atmosphere can be improved considerably by having occasional meetings where employees are encouraged to make positive suggestions on how problems can be overcome, and then acting on those suggestions so that everyone feels more part of a team.

It may be possible to introduce a few office perks. Buying in an on-site massage service is a good way of relieving stress, say giving 10–20 minutes of massage per employee each week. Any expenditure on encouraging and helping a workforce to be happy and healthy will surely prove to be cost effective.

Complete the following questionnaire. Be

honest in your responses, giving yourself a score of 0–5 against each question. The resulting total will reveal to you the extent to which stress is a problem in your life. Awareness of this is the first positive step towards dealing with it.

STRESS CHECK AND SCORE LIST	SCORE 0–5
• Are you a poor listener?	
• Do you bite your nails?	
• Do you feel guilty when you relax?	
• Do you grind your teeth?	
• Are you tense, restless and fidgety?	
• Do you have difficulty sleeping?	
• Do you have mood swings?	
• Do you have irregular eating habits?	
• Do you feel you are always being asked to do more than you can cope with?	
• Are you dissatisfied with your job/home life?	
• Do you find it hard to motivate yourself?	
• Do you feel unfit and overweight?	
• Do you have constant worry (money, mortgage, relationships)?	
TOTAL	

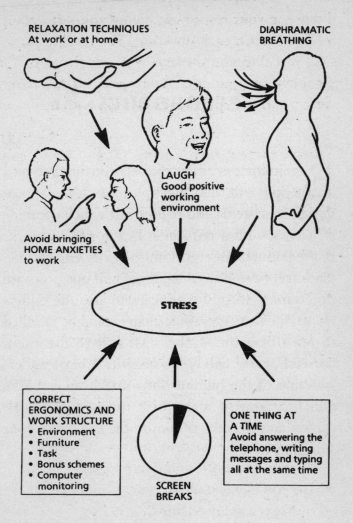

RELAXATION TECHNIQUES
At work or at home

DIAPHRAMATIC
BREATHING

LAUGH
Good positive
working
environment

Avoid bringing
HOME ANXIETIES
to work

STRESS

CORRECT
ERGONOMICS AND
WORK STRUCTURE
• Environment
• Furniture
• Task
• Bonus schemes
• Computer
  monitoring

SCREEN
BREAKS

ONE THING AT
A TIME
Avoid answering the
telephone, writing
messages and typing
all at the same time

51

CHAPTER THREE

Ergonomics

Ergonomics is about the relationship between people and their workplace with the aim of designing systems and equipment which combine efficiency with a reduction in the risk of work-related injury. An ergonomically designed work-place will be to little avail, though, if operators are not trained in how properly to use the equip-ment. The best ergonomic chairs could be installed in an office, but if the staff fail to use them correctly, there will be no benefit. A basic under-standing of the human body and how it works will help you to make best use of your work station, and thereby minimize the chance of your suffering RSI.

SITTING POSTURE

We spend most of the working day sitting in a chair, and then we go home and sit on another chair. I cannot emphasize enough the importance of a good chair, both in the office and the home. It is vital that your chair provides the correct support for your spine, as your spine is the nerve centre through which movement messages are sent to the rest of your body. Persistent wrong sitting posture can result in many problems, such as low back pain, headaches, shoulder ache, sciatica, cervical spondylosis and slipped disc. It is also a contributory factor in RSI. Many of us accept such aches and pains as part of life, but we shouldn't.

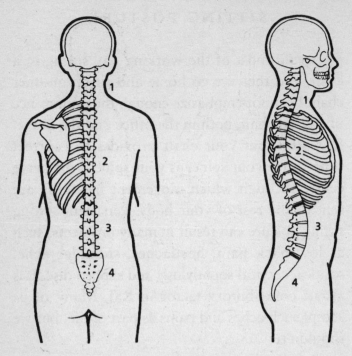

Anatomical structures of and around the spine

As you can see from the diagram of the spine, it has natural curves. It is very important when sitting that these curves are maintained.

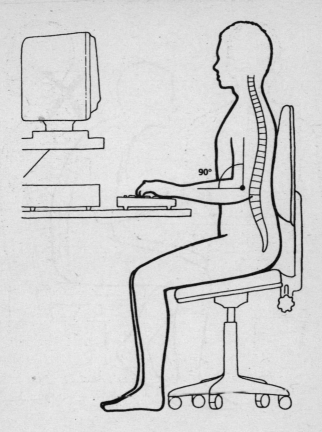

90°

Correct sitting posture

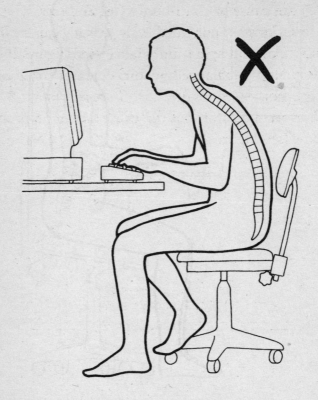

Incorrect sitting posture

Improper leg and foot positions (see Figure 27) can cause or contribute to leg and foot symptoms. Constant one-sided body twisting can create muscular and spinal imbalance (see Figure 28). Assuming unbalanced postures creates strain on your body (see Figure 29). Slumping may give short-term comfort but can cause long-term problems (see Figure 30).

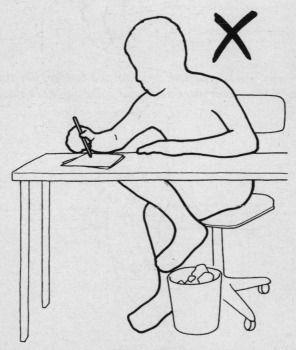

Keep your legs and feet in the proper position. Don't twist them like this

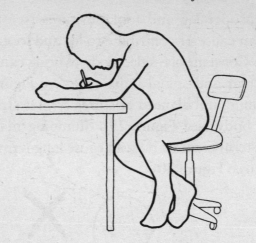

If you sit for long periods in a twisted fashion like this it puts an unnecessary strain on your spine and back muscles

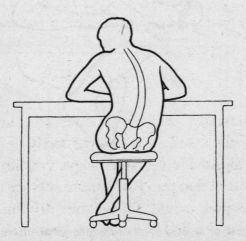

Bad posture puts strain on your body

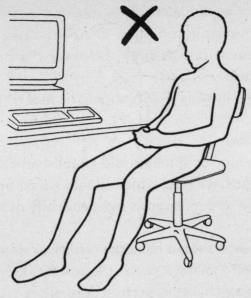

You may get instant relief from slumping in your chair, but you risk future problems if you sit like this all the time

THE RIGHT WAY

A good chair will be designed so that all its components will move independently enabling it to be adjusted to suit your shape, size and height. It is crucial that the chair adjustments are utilized; just as you would adjust your driving seat if someone else had been driving your car and had altered the setting. You do this automatically to prevent an accident! It is essential you do the same for your computer chair—the risk of an accident is just as high, however the onset is insidious.

The following points should be looked for:

Your chair

1. The lumbar spine should be fully supported by the back rest, which should adjust up and down and in and out independently of the seat.

2. The seat should have the facility to slope forward giving a pelvic tilt (a semi automatic rocking facility is preferred, to allow continual movement).

3. The seat depth should comfortably support your legs from hip to knee without putting pressure on the middle of the thigh. The seat should adjust forwards and backwards to accommodate different leg lengths.

4. The chair should adjust in height, from the floor to the seat, to permit you to sit comfortably with your knees bent at about a 90 degree angle.

5. The density of the foam in the seat must be comfortable. There should be enough spring

or give in the chair to support your body and eliminate shock through your spine. However, it should not be so soft that it allows your pelvis to sink into it.

6. There should be a swivel, and a five-castor base to allow the chair to move freely.

7. Arm rests are not absolutely necessary, but in some situations they may be helpful. Their height should be adjustable.

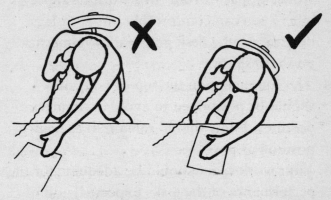

A chair that swivels and rolls saves you having to twist your body

Your desk

1. It is important that the height of your desk allows your forearms to be parallel to the floor while keying.

2. Your elbows should be bent at about 90 degrees or just over and they should be in line with your shoulders.

3. There must be sufficient knee room under the desk, and drawer units should be free-standing so that they can be positioned under an area of the desktop other than that at which you are sitting (e.g. under where you have your in/out trays). I call this 'dead working space'. Your 'live working space' is where you can comfortably put your legs underneath the desk and work symmetrically on the desk top.

4. The equipment on the top of your desk should be positioned to avoid asymmetrical postures. Joints should remain in as neutral a position as possible.

5. Your work space should be adequate for the performance of the tasks expected, and it should be large enough to accommodate all necessary equipment, such as monitor, keyboard, telephone, document holder, etc.

6. The equipment should leave enough room to work comfortably and enable you to rest your hands and arms. [According to the British Standards Institute a desk should be

height adjustable within the range of 660mm to 770mm from floor level. However, if the desk is at a fixed height its surface should be no less than 660mm and no greater than 730mm.]

7. The desktop should be non-reflective to avoid eye strain.

8. An average desk of 28 inches or 710mm will generally be too low for people of 5 ft 9 ins, and those smaller than 5 ft 5 ins will generally require a foot stool. These measurements are dependent on the combination of leg and spine length.

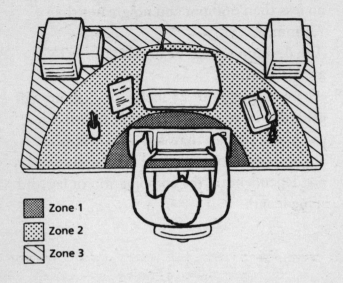

Zone 1
Zone 2
Zone 3

Organize your desk top so that there is space in front of you for immediate tasks, and space for lower-priority items

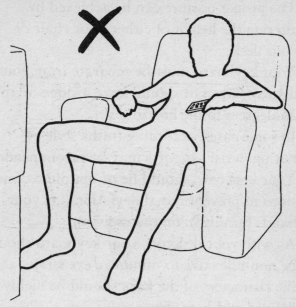

Be aware of good posture both at work and at home, and make it a habit

Your keyboard

1. Your keyboard should be positioned to allow your wrists to be kept parallel to the floor, or sloping slightly downwards.
2. Your wrists should be neutral (not dropped or deviated inwards or outwards) while keying, as this can increase pressure on the carpal tunnel area (see Chapter 1).

3. The proper posture can be achieved by altering the height of either your chair or your desk.

4. Your keyboard must be separate from your display screen (it should have a slope of up to 25 degrees to the horizontal.)

5. In some cases, according to the style of keying, wrist supports may be recommended.

6. Your keyboard should be of optimum dimensions to prevent radial deviation (i.e. your hands turning in on themselves).

7. As with your desktop, your keyboard should be non-reflective to minimize eye strain, and the characters of the keys should be highly defined and kept clean.

8. The keyboard should be situated 3–4 inches from the edge of the desk to allow an area for your wrists when not typing.

Remember, you should leave your desk to go for lunch, and not be eating and dropping crumbs over your keyboard.

Your screen

1. Your screen should be directly in front of you.
2. The body is symmetrically balanced and should not be put under more strain than necessary.
3. The height of the screen should not be above the horizontal plane of your eyes. However, it must be at eye level.
4. The screen should be about an arm's distance away from you whilst sitting correctly in your chair, and it should be able to tilt and rotate, and be separate from the disk drive.
5. The brightness and contrast of the screen should be adjusted in accordance with lighting conditions.
6. The positioning of your screen in relation to natural and artificial light is crucial. Position it at 90 degrees to the light source.
7. There may be circumstances where a visor may be necessary. When buying a visor, be aware that some polarized screen visors can increase reflection even though they may decrease glare.
8. Wearing dark clothing will also reduce reflec-

tion on the screen, and remember to keep your screen clean.

9. The characters on your screen should be clearly defined and about 2–4mm in size.

10. Ensure your screen colours are not causing eye strain, avoid fluorescent multicoloured screens. If uncertain about colours, use monochrome screens.

Lighting and glare

1. Glare and reflection must be minimized.

2. The screen should not be situated in front of the window, as this increases glare, or with the window directly behind, as this will increase reflection.

3. Room lighting must be appropriate for the task, i.e. darker ambient light for computer work and brighter light for paper work.

4. Daylight can be reduced by blinds or tinted glass over the windows.

5. Electric lights should be situated to avoid reflections—uplighters, diffusers and grids will disperse the light.

6. Avoid the colour white as it is the most reflective colour—white walls, white desks,

white paper!

7. Interior glass panelling and glass framed pictures will increase the reflections.

Foot stool

It is necessary that your feet rest comfortably on either the floor or a foot rest. If you use a foot rest it should be positioned on the floor where your feet can comfortably rest on it in a symmetrical fashion. It should not be able to be kicked about underneath the desk. The surface should be non-slip and of a sufficient size to allow your feet to move. The British Standards Institute's recommended size is 450mm long by 350mm wide, with an adjustable angle from 0 to 20 degrees.

Document Holders

These are very helpful when you are keying from copy as they minimize the need for awkward movements of your head and eyes. The ideal document holder is hinged like an angle-poise lamp, and can be situated to the side of the screen at the same height and distance. This also enables the user to distance the text according to size.

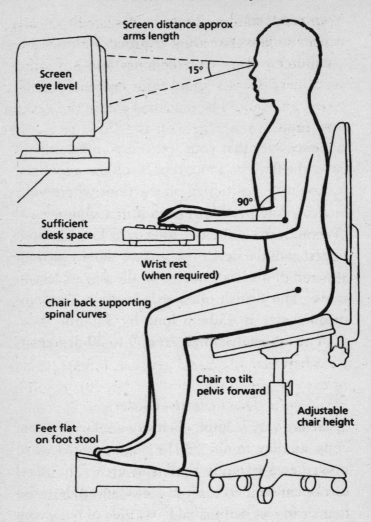

Screen distance approx
arms length

Screen
eye level

15°

90°

Sufficient
desk space

Wrist rest
(when required)

Chair back supporting
spinal curves

Chair to tilt
pelvis forward

Adjustable
chair height

Feet flat
on foot stool

Your work station should be designed to neatly accommodate the cables required for power to computers, printers, telephones and any other machinery. Cables should not encroach on leg space, and should be managed within the desks, and taped or bridged on the floor to avoid tripping.

Temperature and Humidity

A comfortable office temperature should be maintained about 19–23°C (66–73°F). Heat is usually generated by electrical equipment and this needs to be taken account of. If possible switch off machinery at night.

Try to ensure that the relative humidity of the air is between 40 and 60 per cent. Indoor plants or even a bowl of water on the desks are helpful; please ensure they are away from any electrical appliances! You could use a humidifier.

To sum up, the ideal is fully adjustable chairs, desks, screens and keyboards so that equipment can be 'tailored' to suit you personally. Remember that sitting for a fixed time working in front of a computer screen is a high risk occupation.

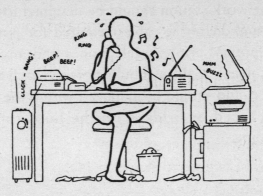

Excessive background noise serves to add to stress levels

Your workplace should be a tidy attractive place, and there should be no unnecessary noise from machinery, unanswered phones, traffic, loud music, as undue mess and distracting noises only serve to increase stress levels. Ensure machines such as faxes and photocopiers are situated somewhere that minimizes their noise distraction. Otherwise try insulating hoods. The ring of the phone should be set at an appropriate volume. Carpeted areas will absorb more noise than linoleum/wood. Windows should be double glazed if there is excess traffic noise outside.

Try completing the following ergonomic audit on your work station to see how it scores.

ERGONOMIC CHECK AND SCORE LIST	SCORE 0–5
CHAIR	
• Height adjustability	
• Backrest adjustability	
• Pelvic tilt or rocking mechanism	
• Seat depth adjustability	
• Five castors and swivel facility	
• Comfort	
DESK	
• Desk size/plan	
• Height adjustability	
• Non-reflective surface	
• Leg room	
• Foot rest provided	
• Document holder provided	
KEYBOARD	
• Keyboard size	
• Non-reflective surface	
• Position (in relation to body)	
• Angle	
• Legible characters	
• Clean	

ERGONOMIC CHECK AND SCORE LIST	SCORE 0–5
SCREEN	
• Screen position (in front)	
• Height (eye level)	
• Distance (arm's length)	
• Reflectivity	
• Swivel and tilt	
• Brightness and contrast adjustments	
• Clean	
LIGHTING	
• Glare	
• Reflections	
• Blinds	
• Overhead electric light grids	
GENERAL	
• Noise level	
• Heat/humidity comfort	
• Air quality/circulation	
• Hazards – cable management/faulty equipment	

What You Should Do If in Pain

The principal aim of this book is to help you avoid RSI, but I realize that you may be reading it already suspecting that you may have some problem. Because of the lack of documented evidence about RSI you could find yourself banging your head against a brick wall when seeking unspecialized medical advice. Many sufferers have found their doctors unhelpful and unsympathetic when they first sought help.

This can be very frustrating, and you may even get to the point where even you begin to feel that it is all in your mind. You know how real your pain is but no one else will believe you. You are not alone, there are many others in the same boat and you must not give up.

The earlier treatment is sought, the quicker your symptoms will be relieved and the less damage will be done. If you are already suffering from recurrent physical aches and pains, please do not dismiss it and take a pain killer. Generally pain killers will only mask the pain and not get rid of the cause. Try not to get worked up and panic as this will only increase your symptoms. Think positively about how you are going to deal with them, and phone one of the contact numbers given. At this stage avoid all activities that aggravate your symptoms, and if work is increasing your symptoms speak to your manager. Not reporting it will only increase the problem for all concerned.

You may find heat and gentle shoulder and neck stretches soothing. Try rolling your shoulders and gently stretching your neck from side to side in a slow relaxed way. Perhaps try using a hot water bottle over areas which ache, or take plenty of hot baths. Heat helps to relax muscle tension. If your arms feel inflamed or swollen do not use heat. You may find ice more soothing. Gentle cardiovascular exercise such as walking (imagine walking like a monkey with long relaxed arms!) and swimming may relieve the symptoms. **Should symptoms become aggravated by any of the above, stop!**

Avoid tense positions. Try to adopt positions of relaxation and lengthening. Lie on the floor or on the bed with a couple of pillows under your knees. Try resting the your head on some books while lying on the floor, to gently stretch your neck. When sitting, avoid slumping in a sofa. Try instead to sit in a reclined position that supports and lengthens your spine.

It is sensible to have your work posture/ ergonomics looked at by a specialist (occupational physiotherapist or ergonomist) as soon as possible to ensure that you are working correctly and that the furniture is appropriate. Do not go back to work and resume any aggravating tasks until this has been done.

If driving, ensure you sit close to the wheel with your elbows down and perhaps supported by a pillow on your lap. Try to relax your shoulders. Once again make sure the seat is supporting your spine. If driving is uncomfortable, avoid it and take public transport until you have seen a therapist.

AVOID:
Carrying heavy shopping
Carrying your handbag on one shoulder (if you must take a bag, ensure it is as light as possible and crossed over your body like a

mail bag, or use a waist purse or rucksac)

Vigorously brushing your teeth (use an electric toothbrush)

Heavy housework such as ironing, hoovering and polishing

Opening tight jars or chopping (try the disabled living shops for domestic aids)

Heavy exercise such as weight-training, racket sports and jogging

Excessive writing (you may find a thicker grip pen helpful)

Playing musical instruments if symptoms are aggravated

Seek the advice of a therapist who works on the mechanics of the body and has some under-standing of RSI and neural tension techniques, such as a physiotherapist, an osteopath, a chiro-practor, a massage therapist, an Alexander Technique teacher or a shiatsu therapist. We only have one body, and it cannot be replaced, so try to seek some constructive advice as soon as possible. You may find that when you receive treatment your symptoms are volatile and perhaps flare up. Once again do not panic. Speak to your ther-apist and ask advice. The longer you have had symptoms the longer they take to go away. Generally the rate of improvement is slow. Do not expect immediate recovery and do not just give up.

Try to avoid medication, although in some circumstances anti-depressants, anti-inflammatories and pain-killers may help.

You may find that some of the alternative therapies can help to reduce your symptoms—such as acupuncture, Chinese medicine and hypnosis. These therapies are holistic in their approach and often seem to help sufferers.

Useful Addresses

Here are some addresses and telephone numbers which may be helpful in your search for a diagnosis and treatment.

Chalmers Mill Consultants UK Ltd t/a
  INTERACT
Premier House
313 Kilburn Lane
London W9 3EG
Tel. 081–968 6633

Specialist physiotherapy and ergonomic workplace assessments

The Chartered Society of Physiotherapy
14 Bedford Row
London WC4 4ED
Tel. 071–242 1941

Physiotherapy—ask for local specialist

The RSI Association
Chapel House
152–156 High Street
Yiewsley
Middlesex UB7 7DD

General information pack

The Musicians and Keyboard Clinic
7 Park Crescent
London W1
Tel. 071–436 5961

Specialist medical advice

The Ergonomic Society
Devonshire House
Devonshire Square
Loughborough LE11 3DW
Tel. 0509 234904

Ergonomic workplace assessments—ask for specialist in screen equipment

FOR GENERAL MASSAGE

The British School of On-Site Massage (Stress-Busters)
48d Camden Street
London NW1
Tel. 071–383 7943

General on-site massage

Colin Erskine
Body Work/massage
Marshall Street Leisure Centre
14–16 Marshall St
London W1V 1LN
Tel. 071–287–1022

General body massage and stretches

The British School of Osteopathy
1–4 Suffolk Street
London SW1
Tel. 071–930–9254

Osteopathy—ask for local specialist

The Society of Teachers in Alexander Technique
(STAT)
20 London House
266 Fulham Road
London SW10 9EL
Tel. 071–351 0828

Specialists in postural re-education

References

Mobilisation of the Nervous System, David S. Butler, Churchill Livingstone, 1991

Fit for Work, Scott Donkin, Kogan Page, 1990

Laughter, The Best Medicine, Robert Holden, Thorsons, 1993

Stress that Motivates, Dru Scott, Kogan Page, 1993

Index